Table of Contents

Bladder Prolapse: Causes, Symptoms, and Treatment Options

Understanding Bladder Prolapse: Causes, Symptoms, Treatment

1. Introduction to Bladder Prolapse

Bladder prolapse falls under a category of conditions that are more commonly referred to as "pelvic organ prolapse". This blanket term is utilized to emphasize the fact that there are many different organs that can experience a change in position in the pelvic cavity. There are many remaining specialists who will only perform this surgery using the open technique. The anterior cutaneous nerve entrapment syndrome is pressure on a nerve in the abdomen that often causes pain. Bladder prolapse has two different types, which are the following: run-of-the-mill cystocele and giant cystocele. Interestingly, the causes of these two types do not differ from one another. In fact, they both arise due to the same common causes. For both types of cystocele, the general causes are bearing down over time, increased abdominal pressure, having had previous vaginal childbirth, and damage to the muscles of the pelvic floor. In terms of symptoms, some individuals may be asymptomatic, but those who do have symptoms are likely to encounter a vaginal bulge or bladder control issues.

In this essay, we will take a closer look at prolapse and the types that are most commonly found in women. In this essay, we will be specifically looking at bladder prolapse. We will be going over the different types of bladder prolapse, what causes them, the symptoms that different individuals may face if they have bladder prolapse, and lastly, the types of treatments that individuals who suffer with bladder prolapse may receive, which includes both surgical and non-surgical treatments.

2. Anatomy of the Bladder and Pelvic Floor

The pelvic floor muscles work with certain connective tissues (fascia) of fine threads that connect the front and back of the pelvic skeleton. Together, the muscles and fascia create a stable sling that carries the weight of the bladder and other pelvic organs. If the pelvic floor muscles are too weak to carry this load, the fascia can give way under the load. The deterioration of the pelvic floor supporting fascia seems to be the initial developmental path of the bladder that sags into the vagina.

The bladder is a hollow, balloon-like organ in the pelvis that holds urine. Its function is to store urine and, when it's the right time, to empty easily and completely. The pelvic floor is a series of muscles and connective tissues that form a sling across the opening of the pelvis and support the organs (including the bladder) within it. These muscles have many diverse functions, including the support of organs, sexual function, and sphincteric function, which help keep continence. The digestive and urinary tract openings travel through these muscles to exit the body.

3. Types of Bladder Prolapse

Urethrocele: This type of bladder prolapse occurs when the urethra drops downward toward the vaginal opening. It may occur by itself or along with other types of prolapse. If you also leak urine when you cough, sneeze, or laugh, it is usually accompanied by a low-lying bladder. Some symptoms may be grouped together, and they may coexist. It is rare to have a urethra that descends without a bladder that goes along with it. In some cases, the urethra protrudes beyond the vaginal opening. If you have a urethrocele, your doctor may want to check you for problems urinating. To do this, they may ask if you have any of the following symptoms: a weak or slow urinary stream, inability to completely empty your bladder.

- Grade 1: Sometimes known as mild prolapse, the bladder has descended within the vagina but does not stick out through the opening. - Grade 2: The bladder is much closer to the vaginal opening. But just like grade 1, the bladder still has not fully begun to stick out through the opening of the vagina. - Grade 3: Also known as advanced prolapse, the bladder can very easily bulge out of the vaginal opening without even having to strain. It may also be possible for the bladder to stick out only when forced to. - Occult: This is a hidden type of prolapse. In this stage, the bladder is located lower within the pelvis than it should be. This is not visible during a routine speculum exam and requires diagnostic testing to detect it.

There is more than one type of bladder prolapse, and they are all classified by varying stages or grades. Here's a basic breakdown of the different types of this condition:

4. Causes of Bladder Prolapse

Prolapse of the bladder can occur when a female carries any heavy weight on a regular basis, such as when they cough (especially whooping cough), sneeze or laugh, and when more severe forms of prolapsed bladder take place. Cigarette smokers who have chronic cough, for instance, are at increased risk for cystocele. A family background of bladder prolapse could also add to the chance of having prolapse to some degree. Moreover, a genetic connection to tissue integrity, easier access to the healthcare environment, and similar behavior with early repair care are all possible.

When viewed from an outward angle, several underlying causes lead to some form of bladder prolapse to occur. Pregnancy, which causes the pelvic floor muscles and tissue to separate, as well as childbirth, during which the baby moves through the vaginal canal and overstretches or tears the pelvic floor muscles, contribute to the spread of bladder prolapse. The older the patient, the more prone they are to this problem. Bladder prolapse becomes more common with age, which is linked to the body's natural weakening of connective tissues and the gradual loss of estrogen that occurs during menopause. The incidence of totally prolapsed bladder among women increases as they get older. Also increasingly prospective is that the condition will become worse over time.

4.1. Pregnancy and Childbirth

Pregnancy is typically not associated with pelvic organ prolapse (POP), but childbirth is causally aligned as women without vaginal deliveries have the lowest occurrence of POP. The actual damage to pelvic floor support caused by childbirth is poorly understood. The birth canal offers a spectrum of resistance to the cervical dilation process that ranges from almost no resistance to complete resistance. The soft tissues of the body are stretched and retraction tears are common as scarification is experienced. There is little good evidence to support attending risk for the cervical dilation process or the acute damage to the levator ani myo-fascia body closely associated with the process of childbirth. Whether levator injury is a major contributor to the sequelae of prolapse (specific symptoms) is unknown. 'Unassisted delivery' offers some level of spontaneous pelvic floor relaxation to make way for offspring delivery. The overall impact of history vaginal delivery over non-vaginally delivered controls is poorly studied.

Pregnancy and childbirth have been identified as significant causes of bladder prolapse. This problem has been the same over the last 100 years as it is today. The findings have varied, but it has been found that around 22% of women with normal vaginal deliveries later seek care for their bladder prolapse. This point is stressed by the fact that most of the original material for surgery addressed women with childbirth-associated problems: oversized, torn, floppy, and malpositioned reproductive female organs. They are treated no differently today and have large clinical practices.

4.2. Aging and Menopause

As part of the aging process, the body's estrogen production decreases. Estrogen is one of the hormones that help maintain the strength and elasticity of pelvic supportive tissues. As a result of reduced estrogen, the vaginal tissues can become thinner, more fragile, and may produce less natural fluid. Contributory factors to bladder prolapse that likely affect aging women include: anger, muscle severity and tissue tearing, and longstanding increased intra-abdominal pressure (such as years of constipation, heavy lifting, and cough), pregnancy and childbirth, particularly multiple. In a study of 311 Italian women, researchers found that the risk of developing cystocele was significantly related to natural childbirth, longer second stage of labor, and the delivery of the first baby. The risk of developing cystocele increased an estimated 9% for every 7 minutes of longer second stage of labor. Postmenopausal women have been shown to have weaker pelvic tissues than premenopausal women. In a group of 18 healthy postmenopausal volunteers, a significantly reduced yield load (maximum pressure causing rupture) in circumferential descensus, along with overall increased pelvic organ mobility in their pelvises was found compared to a similar group of 9 premenopausal volunteers. In premenopausal women, the ovaries typically produce approximately 20 to 150 picograms (pg) of estradiol (the most common form of estrogen) per milliliter (mL) of blood each day. It is believed that only 10 to 15 pg/mL of estradiol in the blood is needed to maintain pelvic supportive tissues. Postmenopausal women may have a wide range of estrogen levels. One study documented that six of seven postmenopausal women had undetectably low levels of estradiol in their blood and failed to demonstrate signs of systemic estrogen production. Postmenopausal women who are receiving estrogen-replacement therapy involving the low retention vaginal ring, cream, or suppository are actually bathing their prolapsed vaginal wall with the hormone. Another study in vitro showed beneficial effect of vitamin D3 on the tissue quality of vaginal supportive tissues in age-related changes in the postmenopausal woman's body that may contribute to the development of advanced bladder prolapse.

4.3. Chronic Coughing or Heavy Lifting

In prolapse, the bladder descends from its normal midline position between the right and left pelvic bone structure, and presses into the wall of the vagina. When the bladder falls into the vaginal wall, a cystocele is the result. Typically, the bladder and the membrane that holds it, called the vesico-uterine fascia, become dehiscent or torn in the middle of the cystocele, also called the cardinal-uterosacral ligaments, which creates a V-shaped cystocele. It is difficult to definitively say that "X" activity alone causes just a cystocele (other than pregnancy and childbirth), as several occupational and lifestyle activities can weaken the entire pelvic floor through many different mechanisms, resulting in a variety of prolapses. Also, combinations of these activities and associated conditions often occur jointly in women and are likely to contribute to the development of various prolapses in a multiparous woman over her lifetime. Carrying excess weight represents a chronic heavy lifting stress to the pelvic floor, and obesity is another major risk factor for prolapse. High-intensity lifting is particularly exacerbating for incontinence.

Chronic, severe coughing from conditions such as asthma, chronic obstructive pulmonary disease, bronchitis, heavy smoking, and other ailments can strain our pelvic floor, which can contribute to prolapses such as a rectocele, a cystocele, enteroceles, or an apex/cervix vaginal vault prolapse. When the ligaments of the muscles of the pelvic floor are briskly stretched and significantly weakened or damaged, the bladder and other pelvic organs are displaced from their normal anatomical position, resulting in a cystocele. Heavy and repetitive heavy lifting, with or without holding our breath when lifting, particularly during occupational activities, can also weaken the pelvic floor muscles, ligaments, and supporting structures that hold the bladder in its normal position and contribute to prolapse. Occupational lifting can also result in altered passive or intrinsic resting pelvic floor tone and positioning or sitting angle of the pelvis, which can exacerbate prolapse.

5. Risk Factors for Bladder Prolapse

1. Childbirth - The combination of an oversized baby pushing down on the bladder along with the hormonal effects of relaxin can make the vagina temporarily loose after pregnancy, giving the bladder more room to sag. 2. Inappropriate straining during bowel movements - The pelvic and abdominal floor muscles, as well as movement in these structures during straining, can provide support to the pelvic organs. Pushing in a way that does not utilize these muscles or straining too hard with heavy loads can increase intra-abdominal pressure substantially. 3. Chronic cough - More pressure comes down from the bottom of the abdomen when someone has a chronic cough. The usual "pelvic floor" squeeze is not enough to counteract this, leading to more pressure on the pelvic organs.

Risk factors for bladder prolapse include:

Bladder prolapse, also called a cystocele or fallen bladder, can result from a variety of conditions or behaviors. Whenever someone has pressure coming down from above on an organ, it is relatively easy for the organ to get pushed down into the vagina or even to slip between the muscle structures in the pelvis—kind of like a hernia. For the bladder, this might mean that stool is pressing on the uterine wall and downward on the bladder, before which the bladder might even be angling into the vagina, making leakage more likely.

6. Symptoms of Bladder Prolapse

Other symptoms often experienced by those with bladder prolapse include the following: 1. Pelvic pressure, pain, or not feeling well or "more full" as the day progresses, especially when on your feet for long periods of time. 2. Lower back pain: Sometimes this can involve your hips and may go all the way down the legs. 3. Pelvic pain or a feeling of fullness in the pelvic region. 4. Vaginal bleeding or unusual discharge (occasionally seen with severe cases). 5. A mass or something that seems to "fall out" of the vagina.

The most common symptom of bladder prolapse is stress urinary incontinence. This type of incontinence, as detailed above, is leaking that occurs when you are coughing, sneezing, laughing, jumping, or with any activity that increases pressure in the abdomen and puts pressure on the bladder. With bladder prolapse, the neck of the bladder is lower than it should be, causing the angle from the base of the bladder to the urethra to decrease. This can increase the risk of urine leakage. Over time, the ureter may close up to keep urine from flowing backward from the ureter into the kidneys. While this may sound like a "good thing," over time this can cause the bladder to continue to fill even when it is supposed to be empty.

6.1. Urinary Incontinence

Urinary incontinence is the involuntary loss of urine. This is not a disease in its own right, but a serious complication affecting 4 million people in France, particularly those over the age of 50. When it becomes moderate, it considerably affects the lives of the patients who suffer from it, by preventing them from performing activities that bring them into society, working, and causing hygiene and social relations that are difficult to manage. Urinary neurological incontinence appears to respond to sacral neuromodulation (SNM) treatment with different bladder functions. That is why we propose to report the efficiency and tolerance of SNM in terms of the different types of urinary incontinence and the severity of these patients.

The first important symptom of bladder prolapse or cystocele (anterior prolapse) is urinary incontinence, especially when standing and walking. The bladder and urethra require the support of the pubocervical fascia, as well as the levator-urethra muscle. Stress incontinence, urinary incontinence in bladder prolapse, is characterized by urine losses of variable but generally small volume. It occurs when intra-abdominal pressure rises in the absence of detrusor contraction (initially or temporarily). Because the causes of urinary losses that begin with stress incontinence rarely stop there, a systematic research of the two basic mechanisms is also recommended. However, isolated stress incontinence is by definition rare and generally resolves due to hypoestrogenism. Because the organ that can lose its support is the bladder, urinary disorders are the main symptom, encouraging further discussion of these alone, with email the data from the literature.

6.2. Pelvic Pressure or Pain

The importance of accurate diagnosis of bladder prolapse cannot be overemphasized when considering these discomfort symptoms. In some cases, chronic cervicitis, pelvic pain syndrome, urethral syndrome, vestibulitis, coccygodynia, hemorrhoids, scratch anorectum, and anal fissure are incorrectly diagnosed when pelvic organ prolapses actually account for these presenting symptoms. Great care needs to be taken about possible neuropathic or urologic involvement, and dedicated investigations, such as anorectal manometry, electrical stimulations, and electromyography should be used to reach a proper diagnosis. Furthermore, organ prolapse patients with no urogynecologic symptoms have a higher prevalence of rectoanal symptoms (e.g., chronic constipation), fecal incontinence, and anal incontinence, anorectal pain, since impairment of pelvic floor muscle support and enteroceles also account for these symptoms.

The second most common symptom of bladder prolapse is experiencing pelvic pressure or pain. Because this area of the body is involved in so many daily activities, discomfort in the pelvic area can dramatically reduce one's quality of life and disrupt daily activities for those experiencing it. The pain and pressure can either be constant or intermittent, and some women notice it more in the evenings after a long day spent standing. Often, women will note the most pain when standing for long periods of time, picking up heavy items, or after a prolonged period of sitting, particularly on a hard surface.

7. Diagnosis of Bladder Prolapse

Imaging tests can help healthcare providers diagnose bladder prolapse. You may have an MRI, a scan in which pictures are taken to examine the muscles and tissues. You may also have a type of CT scan that uses X-rays and a computer to create pictures of the bladder. Imaging can help show the severity and full extent of your prolapse, and it can guide planning for treatment. Accurately diagnosing your prolapse will help your healthcare provider develop the best treatment plan for your needs. A physical exam is worth a thousand tests. If you are seeking a definitive diagnosis and a treatment plan that truly cares for your concerns, consider scheduling a consultation at The Center for Innovative GYN Care.

How is bladder prolapse diagnosed? Your healthcare provider will begin by discussing your symptoms and medical history. A physical exam will be performed. If you are not menstruating, your healthcare provider may perform a pelvic exam when you are lying down or standing up. These positions can make it easier to diagnose prolapse. If you are menstruating, your health care provider will probably only perform an exam while you are lying down. During the pelvic exam, the healthcare provider will identify the type and severity of the prolapse. Your provider will also look for other problems and be sure that your bladder, bowel, and other pelvic organs are working normally.

7.1. Physical Examination

Observation in the standing and lying patients before palpating at rest. This is an important component of examination in order to differentiate anatomic components of pelvic organ prolapse from vaginal bulging due to increased laxity or atrophy/defect. This is when attentive examination can be done in order to see if cystocele or rectocele reduces or disappears when prolapse is reduced by retracting it using hand. Observation of the bladder on the hand placed on the pelvis during standing to assess for bladder signal. Observation of the anterior vaginal wall displacement during the Valsalva. Palpation perhaps during the delivery of the test dose of local anesthetic.

Exercise 1: Intake and micturition observation and palpation

The physical examination evaluates the resting position of the bladder and urethra. It also assesses muscle function and structure. Used for assessment techniques, tactile examination includes visual inspection, comparison of the position of the bladder and urethra during a Valsalva maneuver, and repeated palpation of the lower urethra and the area near the urethral orifice. Quantification is essential, as it will make the result precise and will help in the follow-up.

7.2. Imaging Tests

Magnetic Resonance Vaginography - This is a novel investigation wherein the MRI scan is done during Valsalva maneuver, which is needed for fixation of the bladder in its anatomic position. It will give an idea about the depth of rectal prolapse and other pelvic floor abnormalities, which will aid in the decision-making related to the corrective pelvic surgery. This is cost-effective, and it also identifies previously undiagnosed lesions in the urachal fold and enterocele and would be helpful in deciding the line of management.

Magnetic Resonance Imaging (MRI): The MRI imaging technique uses a combination of a powerful magnet, radio waves, and a computer to produce the detailed images of the internal body organs. The procedure uses an MRI scanner to detect the anatomical changes in the structure between abdomen and vagina, the bladder filled with saline, uterus and rectum in the stomach area.

Ultrasound: This is an imaging technique that uses sound waves to visualize the structure of the internal body organs. The ultrasound imaging helps in visualizing the structure between abdomen and vagina including the bladder.

The imaging tests help to identify the anatomical changes and to confirm the presence of prolapse. The following are the imaging tests used by doctors:

8. Treatment Options for Bladder Prolapse

In general, there are two possible treatment options for women with a prolapsed bladder: conservative and surgical. Conservative treatment involves education about ways to manage symptoms without opting for surgical correction. This could include dietary and lifestyle changes. Also, it can include the use of a pessary to help hold the prolapse in place. A pessary can be an option to help decrease pressure symptoms of a bladder prolapse. A pessary is a rubber or silicone device that fits into the vagina to support the pelvic organs. It is necessary to see a provider once every three to six months for a routine pessary check. If it is difficult to do this, surgical treatment for the prolapse is often a better option. Some women without bothersome symptoms choose to live with a prolapse and do not seek any treatment.

There are many different treatment options for a prolapsed bladder. Conservative treatments include safe and effective physical therapy and pessaries, which are devices fitted into the vagina to give support. Sometimes a combination of these treatments is best. Surgery, if needed, depends on the extent and location of the prolapse, as well as the woman's goals. The unique need for treatment, as well as the selection of a treatment modality, varies greatly between individuals. Pelvic floor physical therapy can be effective for all women with a prolapsed bladder but may not provide long-term benefit for all.

8.1. Conservative Treatments

Be careful in attempts to perform the exercises by yourself, as incorrect performance may make your POP worse. Improper exercises done without supervision may also leave you with a sensation of "heaviness" in the vagina, which may be confused for a worsening of the prolapse. Strong pelvic floor muscles provide support to the vaginal wall muscles and will make the vagina feel stronger, thus avoiding the sensation.

Lifestyle Changes While initial findings of the cause of pelvic wall conditions point to genetic factors, lifestyle habits can affect the severity and rate of prolapse and symptoms a person has. These include: • Performing manual work for 20 or more hours per week increases the risk of prolapse • If normal weight gain in pregnancy occurs, the incidence of prolapse after pregnancy is about the same for "vaginal delivery" and "Cesarean section" groups • Constipation and straining at stool should be avoided as it weakens the pelvic floor muscles, including the muscle support around the bladder replanting of the posterior vaginal wall. Hormone replacement therapy to reduce the risk of Pelvic floor exercises are the "rehabilitation" aspect of prolapse treatment that will result in increasing the strength and function of the pelvic floor muscles. The pelvic floor muscles help give a person control over functions like bowel and bladder continence and support. The exercises can be beneficial for both POP surgery candidates, as well as women who do not want to have surgery.

The few conservative treatments that have been studied include: • Making changes to lifestyle habits in order to decrease the risk and severity of prolapse • Pelvic floor muscle exercises (Kegels) • Use of vaginal pessaries to "lift the bladder off the front wall of the vagina" through the use of a device and prevent discomfort from "falling out."

(2) A healthcare practitioner trained in the treatment of pelvic floor conditions (such as a Physical Therapist, Nurse Continence Advisor, Nurse Practitioner, Gynecologist, Urogynecologist, or Urologist) should guide you through treatment to ensure that you perform the treatment correctly and the treatment is right for you.

(1) If you do not have bothersome symptoms or may want to avoid surgery, even if bothered by symptoms, options for conservative management of POP exist. The primary goals of conservative management are to have good bowel and bladder control and to improve the quality of life in performing daily activities. Conservative options are non-invasive or entail non-surgical approaches towards the management of POP.

8.2. Surgical Interventions

8.2.2. Contraindications Open abdominal procedures for the treatment of bladder prolapse are generally reserved for more advanced or surgically challenging cases. Patients with a history of extensive pelvic radiation that are not candidates for tissue morcellation are best served with abdominal approaches. Marked adhesions from previous surgery may also limit surgical dissection and make the risk of abdominal entry higher for an open approach. Patient emergency urgent surgery indicated with the possibility of complex vaginal repair and vaginal diversion (ureteric catheterization, cystostomy, or in our case of long narrow vagina, performing a colpotomy 6–7 cm from the posterior fornix must be done in suitable conditions with the third arm of Da Vinci (Table 3). The chosen access to apply will be transabdominal if previous CS or TLSO or to perform laparoscopic technique if no previous abdominal operation.

8.2.3. Trigone-sparing vesicovaginal fistula repair with abdominal approach (open or robotic urgent repair).

1) Vaginal hysterectomy and anterior colporrhaphy. There are only a few absolute contraindications to vaginal repair, including patients who have severe radiation damage to the paravaginal fascial attachments and total anatomic dehiscence. New data are suggesting that the preoperative use of 200 mg of Misoprostol 12 to 24 h preoperatively might result in more adequate operating conditions as the bladder can be best mobilized in a filled state. The

placement of biologic or synthetic mesh may decrease the rates of recurrent apical vault prolapse. Like other nonabsorbable biomaterials, vaginal retropubic TVM (TransVaginal Mesh) placement may be considered in a select patient population concerned about recurrent prolapse, provided that the patient understands and accepts the risks and benefits associated with this procedure.

8.2.1. Open Vaginal

Surgical options for the treatment of bladder prolapse can be broken down into open vaginal procedures, minimally invasive vaginal procedures, laparoscopic and robotic-assisted procedures, or open abdominal procedures. The choice of procedure is dependent on patient factors, surgeon preference, and the degree of organ prolapse. The following is a summary of the procedures, increasing in aggressiveness.

9. Prevention Strategies

One means of lowering the risk of prolapsed bladder is to conserve and improve the health of a woman's pelvic floor. There are preventative steps to minimize the impact of risk factors associated with prolapsed bladders. For example, pursuing patience when attempting to relieve a bowel movement and taking time during urination to entirely empty the bladder is not expected to reduce the risk of developing a prolapsed bladder. While it isn't uncommon for chronic pulmonary disease to be associated with a chronic cough, medical management can certainly heal some of the deteriorating conditions that elicit a blaring cough. If a woman appears to be at risk of developing a prolapsed bladder, she may be able to discover the repetitive movements and straining efforts that may be the source of her stress incontinence. If the cough is effectively managed by a doctor, it can reduce the risk of developing a prolapsed bladder.

1. Losing/maintaining weight 2. Avoiding straining constipation 3. Feminine hygiene 4. Treatment of chronic coughing 5. Avoiding repetitive activities

When it comes to preventing a prolapsed bladder arising from the tissue, there are many actions a person can take to stop constriction. Ultimately, a prolapsed bladder defines a condition that arises when muscles and tissues support the person's bladder. There is an abundance of preventative steps; though, as it stands, there is no way to guarantee prevention. The best preventative strategy includes safely harnessing the necessary bodily functions and the maintenance of one's overall health. Since bladder descents often occur due to weakened or damaged pelvic muscles, women wishing to avoid prolapsed bladder can follow these lifestyle changes:

10. Living with Bladder Prolapse

To describe, living with bladder prolapse was defined as meaning living with the mental and emotional aspects of non-impaired well-being and comfort and disruption of normal activities, interfering with fellowship, family, and work roles. Changes in form, function, role, and lifestyle adapt grammar. It affects the living environment and well-being of the individual, family, and the workplace as well. Bladder prolapse uterero laps may also jeopardize one's view of oneself from the physical sense of dependence or pigeon with restrictions, by causing the appearance of counseling and disturbing a coma. Individuals evaluated their own situation in bladder prolapse, in comparison to normal joy, compliance, or a sense of frustration when comparing the same condition with individuals suffering from other ailments of hospitalized chronic illness.

Independent of the extent and nature of the prolapse, living with bladder prolapse can be frustrating, distressing, and often inconvenient. Urine leakage and the persistent need to empty the bladder can be demoralizing and particularly inconvenient for social and work situations. Some individuals diagnosed with bladder prolapse decline surgical intervention for fear of a transient surgical adverse event, having to take time off work or recuperating, while others may not be willing to stop their medication. Some individuals worry about further loss of condition, size, weight, pain, nausea, stress, physical labor, the need for a special diet, proprietary costs, complications, or known side effects of medications or something that I consume casually when the adjustment of the treatment status or weight of my treatment will be known. In some cases, individuals may wish to explore alternatives to drug therapy use, for example, Botox injections for overactive bladder where efficacy is proven to occur and the unfortunate event is called urinary while others cannot afford treatment. The costs of all of this include overweight, urinary health, and quarters and local time; all are contributors to the individual's decision to engage in or continue therapy.

11. Research and Innovations in Bladder Prolapse Management

Continued research efforts in the area of bladder prolapse focus on a wide range of subjects, from anatomical and biomechanical investigation, investigator-initiated trials on modifications of established methods, identifying some of the physiological consequences of urinary incontinence, rectal emptying function, bladder pressure at the time of emptying and various spaces and diameters including the bladder itself or on other aspects of prolapse. Anatomical and biomechanical studies are scientifically interesting with clinical relevance. You can use the findings to develop and evaluate new therapeutic approaches and improve the dialogue with patients about their prolapse and any possible treatments. Ongoing research is also focused on the management of stress urinary incontinence, a common concomitant disorder in many women with prolapse and due to the size of this problem, major research efforts are needed to gain better understanding of the influences of different native and mesh-population characteristics, surgical procedures and confounding factors.

The area of PVD well known among women is the groin. The anterior vaginal wall prolapse with associated bladder descent leads towards an abnormal and pronounced narrowing of the (hence-developed) urogenital hiatus. Basing treatment on anatomic location of prolapse is also not bettering POP management. A systematic review suggests that individual POP stage of a woman neither accurately predicts baseline symptoms nor changes symptoms after failed or successful prolapse or anti-incontinence surgery. Any attempt to categorize POP by premorbid continence status is also not feasible. Thus identifying an etiologic pathway will make incontinence surgery tailored anatomically and functionally in a reliable, subgrouped manner. Findings from our study have implications for research and developing new methods to treat PVD and, currently, there are no data to support a particular intervention for PVD or UGPFI.

Bladder Prolapse: Causes, Symptoms, and Treatment Options

1. Introduction to Bladder Prolapse

A prolapsed bladder is a condition that results from the weakening of vaginal and pelvic muscles that happens over time due to various things, but primarily due to pregnancy and trauma from vaginal labor and delivery. In a prolapsed bladder, the tissues and structures close to or around the bladder fall out of place, sometimes bulging into or outside of the vagina and creating a sensation of heaviness or pressure. There are varying degrees and levels of each of the different types of bladder prolapse, from less severe to more severe. They start at stage one and advance to stage four.

A prolapsed bladder, or cystocele, happens when the bladder descends into the vagina due to the weakening or stretching of the muscles and tissues in the pelvic floor. There are many variations from mild to severe, most likely stemming from the natural wear and tear of birth followed by age, gravity, lifestyle factors, or some combination of those. Some level of prolapse is reported by about 50% of women by age 55, with many of these women noticing nothing or only mild symptoms. There are four stages to standard types of cystocele prolapse (anterior vaginal wall prolapse): Enterocele prolapse is when the top of the vagina falls toward the anus (posterior vaginal wall prolapse); a uretherocele is when the urethra protrudes. Visceral prolapse was the previous term used to describe these conditions that now are more accurately called cystocele, enterocele, and uretherocele.

1.1. Definition and Overview

This condition, also called cystocele, occurs in adult women and is particularly common as women age. An understanding of the complex interactions between the tissues, muscles, ligaments, and other anatomical sites that support the organs of the pelvis is required to understand the causes of pelvic organ prolapse, including cystocele and related conditions such as rectocele and uterine prolapse. Knowing the signs, symptoms, and risk factors of a bladder prolapse is important for being able to address it adequately. This article also provides an overview of diagnosis and the available treatment options, including home remedies. Avoiding urinary infections is a vital part of preventing the problem.

Bladder prolapse is a type of pelvic organ prolapse. It occurs when soft tissues and ligaments that hold the bladder in place stretch or weaken and no longer provide adequate support. This causes the bladder to bulge downward and out of the body through the vagina. While mild cases of prolapse can be minimally symptomatic, more severe cases can cause the entire bladder - or even organs more distally than the bladder such as the uterus or rectum - to move through the vaginal opening.

Bladder prolapse: Definitions and overview

1.2. Types of Bladder Prolapse

A second form of bladder prolapse is known as a posterior cystocele. A pouch of the lining of the rectum, known as anterior rectocele, usually forms along with posterior cystocele. This causes the anterior wall of the rectum to protrude lower into the vagina. Proctocystocele occurs when the rectum descends along with the bladder into the vagina. The urethrocele is a rare form of bladder prolapse defined by a prolapse of the midurethra. It may also appear in cases of cystocele. If the bladder prolapses directly behind the uterus, this is known as a high-grade bladder prolapse. This type of prolapse has already been resolved. Estrogen treatment is not necessary in order to remove it. In an effort to diagnose the various varieties of bladder prolapse, a healthcare provider may employ a particular examination called a pelvic examination.

Bladder prolapse manifests in various forms. These different types of bladder prolapse are based on where the bladder has descended to within the pelvis. The most common type of bladder prolapse is called cystocele. A cystocele occurs when the front wall of the vagina collapses into the vaginal canal and causes the bladder to descend. Occasionally, the urethra (the tube draining from the bladder to the outside of the body) will also be involved in a cystocele. Urethral prolapse is what we call it when the urethra bulges out of the urinary opening as a result of a cystocele. Urethral prolapse, or the protrusion of the female urethra, can also happen on its own. This condition is generally not noticeable and is only diagnosed when the urethra has fallen considerably.

2. Anatomy and Physiology of the Pelvic Floor

The bladder sits very neatly on top of these muscles. With both ends tethered, the body of the bladder does not drop when the pelvic floor muscles disappear - truly, get lost, such as graves people. Or these muscles might never have grown. All the causes of cystoceles and bladder prolapse have to do with the anatomy - where the ligaments are. The woman with a grade one cystocele has a cervix bladder where the six o'clock position is very low. This is pushing the bladder base down toward the kitchen floor. At grade two, the cervix bladder modifies slope, so that the six o'clock is straight back. At grade three, the cervix has disappeared into the vault of the vagina. Overall, however, it's still the six o'clock position that is the cause of the grade of cystocele.

The smaller muscles of the pelvic floor act as a hammock or gores among the pubic symphysis and the coccyx. They hold the rod into place, they cup the earthenware plate that is the pelvic inlet, stopping anything falling from the cavity above, and they form a mini-trampoline for when you bounce. The partition between the colon and uterus and the vagina are like the mesh on a trampoline. They help stop downward bulge.

The pelvic floor is a whole series of muscles and ligaments situated below the pelvis and is directly related to bladder support and function.

2.1. Structure and Function of the Pelvic Floor Muscles

The pelvic floor muscles act to: (1) Close off the pelvic outlet, i.e., the urethra, vagina, and anus; (2) Support the internal organs, namely the bladder in women and the rectum in men; (3) Control intra-abdominal pressure, which changes according to the task being carried out. This, in turn, affects the closing function of the urethra, vagina, and anus. Urethral closure helps prevent urinary incontinence, while anal closure prevents gas and fecal incontinence. In women, a primary support mechanism for the urethra is the levator ani muscle. If central support is compromised, it may lead to urethral hypermobility and GO, resulting in SUI.

The enclosed circle of the perineum muscles joins the pelvic floor muscles, but not all authors take the same view. The pelvic floor helps control intra-abdominal pressure with the deep, stabilizing fibers of these muscles working in conjunction with the transversus abdominis.

The pelvic floor muscles envelop the pelvis and resemble a net of muscles that stretch between the ischial tuberosities and the sacrum, pubic rami, pubic symphysis, and coccyx. These muscles also stretch across the obturator foramen laterally. Barry and Kropf wrote extensively about the pelvic floor in the fourth edition of Gray's Anatomy. St Clair-Thomas, in comparing this edition to the first edition of the book, noted changes in our understanding, including the fact that the pelvic floor is more intensely muscular than previously thought.

2.2. Role in Bladder Support

The bladder also has supports from below provided by an area in the fascia, or "protective and encasing fascia," called the "pubourethral ligaments." Beneath that is a sheet of fibrous tissue that crosses back and forth called the "arcus tendineus fascia pelvis" or ATFP that cradles the bladder. Beneath this is a fabric of muscles that form the pelvic floor. Supporting these supports is a great deal of connective tissue. One can imagine these layers like multiple layers in a trifle dessert jelly bean that provide texture and structure as a thick creamy consistency is poured spoon by spoon on top. This connective tissue is made up of sheets of longitudinal and diagonal tissue made of collagen that work best when the muscle sheets, ligaments, or fascia are connected to their anchor at one end and the back of a bony bone at the other, as it provides a tension-based alignment of the fibers giving the tissue power and resilience coupled with flexibility.

The pelvic floor plays an essential role in supporting the organs of the pelvis, including the bladder. It acts as a sling that wraps around the organs, cordoning off the cavernous area within the pelvis. The urethra, which is also partially encased by the pubococcygeous muscle or PC muscle (a critical part of the pelvic floor), serves to channel urine away from the bladder and prevents leaking. To keep the urinary bladder from sliding out of place, there are two vertical extensions of the muscular wall of the vagina called "ligaments" that anchor the bladder to the bony wall of the pelvis. The top of the organ is separate from the vaginal wall and is only loosely surrounded by additional layers of connective tissue and the peritoneum (a layer that covers and is the deepest part of the inside of the pelvis).

3. Causes and Risk Factors of Bladder Prolapse

Subsequently, as a woman ages, the muscles and supportive tissues surrounding the bladder may gradually weaken over time due to the normal hormonal changes of menopause, the aging process itself, and the repeated stretching and straining that can occur in some women as a result of conditions like chronic constipation. Postmenopausal women who have had children are at the highest risk of developing the symptoms of a prolapsed vagina and uterus, called vaginal vault or uterine prolapse. Women who continue to take hormone replacement therapy after menopause have a slightly lower risk of developing a vaginal prolapse.

There are several risk factors that can predispose someone to having a prolapsed bladder. Risk factors related to pregnancy include older age at first pregnancy, delivery of a large infant, the use of forceps or vacuum during attempted vaginal delivery, and multiple pregnancies. There are several anatomical reasons why pregnancy and childbirth might predispose to a prolapsed bladder in women. The first cause is the trauma to the supportive connective tissue that occurs during childbirth. The second is the direct damage to the nerves and muscles that occurs during childbirth, which may lead to chronic increases in abdominal pressure.

A prolapsed bladder, or cystocele, occurs when the bladder droops down from its usual position and pushes into the front wall of the vagina. Bladder prolapse commonly occurs in association with other forms of pelvic organ prolapse, including uterine prolapse and urethral prolapse. The causes of a prolapsed bladder fall under two main categories: pregnancy and childbirth and chronic increased pressure within the abdomen and pelvis. Direct causes may include conditions such as obesity, having a long-term chronic cough, or heavy lifting.

3.1. Pregnancy and Childbirth

There is a lot of extra weight and pressure put onto the pelvic floor muscles and connective tissues, which hold all the pelvic organs in place. The movement of the baby from above the pelvic floor muscles down through the vaginal birth canal (around the rectum and lower back area) can cause further stretching of the pelvic floor muscles and ligaments. Pushing during childbirth increases the pressure, pushing the womb and vagina further down and expanding the vaginal canal to help allow the baby to pass out. After childbirth, swelling occurs around the baby's head, and as the tissues start to heal, scar tissue is formed, which forces the vagina to stretch out more. When the tissues heal and scar tissue forms, the vaginal lining will usually stretch back to its original size with time, especially if sex is gentle and not possible until the doctor has said it's okay. The bottom part of the uterus is joined to the upper end of the front wall of the vagina, where it can become detached when giving birth. Damage to the front wall of the vagina or the connective tissues from giving birth, if not healed properly, can cause the bladder to sag and prolapse. The damage to the front wall of the vagina or the connective tissues during childbirth may not cause a woman to notice problems for many months or years after childbirth.

During pregnancy, the skin and muscles all over a woman's body stretch and soften, becoming more flexible as the body loosens up to make room for the growing baby. The ligaments holding the pelvic organs in place become more elastic, as do the connective tissues, and there is potential for them to stretch and cause prolapse. The growing baby presses down on the abdominal and pelvic organs at the front and back of the pelvis. If the pelvic floor muscles and connective tissues are weak, organs in the pelvis may be pushed down and cause a prolapse. Hormones are also released to soften and loosen the connective tissues in the body to prepare the mother for birth.

3.2. Aging and Menopause

A study on young women aged 18-39 found a prolapse incidence of 3%. In young women, trauma, obesity, increased abdominal pressure, and decreased estrogen production during menopause are factors that can cause prolapse. Pregnancy history and childbirth are risk factors for prolapse. The incidence is reported to increase by 40% after one childbirth and up to 50% after two births. But, the exact cause of prolapse during or after childbirth is not clearly defined. Damage to the structure of the pelvic floor muscles (PFM) may occur. Pregnancy is also associated with the development of prolapse. Hormonal changes associated with pregnancy and delivery can lead to laxity in pelvic joint tissue. A study in Oslo, Norway, found that parity had an independent effect on bladder prolapse in both non-Asian and Asian subjects. While one study in Baltimore, U.S., found no significant relationship between parity and organ prolapse.

Menopause can occur as early as 40, while the average age is 52. During menopause, a woman's period stops, indicating the end of reproductive capacity. Menopause causes a decrease in estrogen hormone levels, which has many physical effects on a woman's body. About 80% of women experience menopausal stage symptoms while in stage 3 or ovarian failure. Menopause occurs when stage 3 starts and ends when stage 4 begins. A study in the U.S. found that the occurrence of prolapse was higher at the time of evaluation in postmenopausal women. This is due to physiological aging and hormonal factors that influence the strength and elasticity of the pelvic tissues. The force due to pressure that causes prolapse worsens due to the loss of urethral pressure both at rest and during activity. Bladder prolapse is less common in premenopausal women and young women, representing only 20% of all situations.

3.3. Chronic Constipation and Straining

When a woman pushes hard to have a bowel movement, the best diagnostic evidence of the anatomic distension (with or without muscle defects) of the pelvic floor is to note a ballooning of the posterior and/or anterior vaginal wall. The mechanics is simple. Just like a balloon in which a hole in one end can cause a bulge in the other, so can straining to move stool in the rectum cause descent of the other pelvic organs against the pelvic floor. Supplying laxatives or other products to increase stool bulk may alleviate symptoms but nevertheless stress the pelvic support structures to the same degree. Bladder prolapse and overactive morbidity may improve crime management; even after surgery for incontinence, the genital prolapse increases the long-term risk of stress incontinence. For in the detonation go out the through he to them.

Chronic constipation is one of the major contributing risk factors for women who develop bladder prolapse. Not all constipation activities strain the pelvic organs in a damaging way, but straining with defecation can contribute to the development of pelvic floor problems. A wide range of pelvic floor disorders coexist in women with constipation caused by straining. Simply holding the stool with no movement or discomfort is not expected to have significant effects. The downward (and sideways) "angulation" between the rectum and the anus that is necessary to have a normal bowel movement causes mechanical stress to the pelvic floor, especially if sustained over a long time. This anatomical layout is a contributing factor, but there appear to be hereditary factors that limit the ability of the pelvic floor muscles to endure these forces. The biggest causes are childbirth and genetic susceptibility, but considerable chronic straining contributes to bladder prolapse as part of a range of pelvic floor organs.

How Chronic Constipation and Straining Affect the Bladder

4. Signs and Symptoms of Bladder Prolapse

Conversely, it is important to understand the symptoms of bladder prolapse across various stages, as it can alter overall treatment strategies. Recognizing symptoms prior to significant advancement of the condition can provide less invasive treatment options, reducing the need for surgical interventions. Bladder prolapse is associated with several signs and symptoms, as detailed below. Bladder prolapse is associated with a decrease in life quality and a variety of physical symptoms. Proper diagnosis and treatment can lead to improved quality of life, reduced comorbidities, and a greater well-being overall. Patients with bladder prolapse have urinary incontinence, urgency, and frequency. Pelvic problems such as dyspareunia, pelvic pressure or pain, and visible bulge in the genitalia are also common in patients. In most instances, bladder prolapse is due to musculoskeletal deficiencies, leading to frailty in the supportive tissues of the female genitalia. Treatments such as pelvic physical therapy or bladder training can help to improve these symptoms. However, in cases where conservative therapy options have failed or for patients who are not interested in trying them, surgery may be an alternative.

One of the most noticeable symptoms of bladder prolapse is urinary incontinence, or the loss of bladder control. This is not only uncomfortable, but it can be embarrassing and disrupt daily life. Urinary incontinence leads to dribbling and constant moisture. Another common thing women will notice if they have bladder prolapse is acute pelvic pressure or pain. This often feels like "everything is coming down" on them, causing a unique discomfort in the pelvic region. When the bladder creates a bulge inside the vagina, this is called cystocele. It can be uncomfortable and can also sometimes lead to a visible bulge hanging out from the vagina. Not all women are able to see the vaginal bulge, but many cystoceles can be felt by a doctor during the female pelvic examination. When people have pain or discomfort in the vagina or a bulge that is landing out of the vagina, that can also be part of a bladder prolapse. When women have full thickness prolapse, or when prolapse comes through the entrance to the vagina, this is called eversion. Bladder prolapse does not cause eversion alone - it agglomerates with a variety of different varieties of prolapse at the same time. Most of the time, eversion is accompanied by rectocele (falling of the rectum), vaginal vault prolapse (falling of the vagina in women who have had a hysterectomy), or enterocele (herniation of the small intestines).

4.1. Urinary Incontinence

Stress incontinence is one of the most common symptoms of cystocele. It happens because the bladder is no longer in its normal position. Normally, when a person coughs or sneezes, the tension in the vaginal wall helps squash the urethra. This squirt of urine is eliminated. But if the bladder sags or drops into the front wall of the vagina, the relationship between the bladder, urethra, and vaginal wall is changed. Urine escapes when pressure on the body rises. Urge incontinence (detrusor overactivity) is another type of incontinence that can occur with cystocele. In some women, the tension or the hanging of the bladder into the vagina makes the bladder very irritable and causes it to contract unexpectedly, causing unexpected urinary loss. Some people with urge incontinence may experience a urinary frequency called urgency.

The primary symptom of bladder prolapse is urinary incontinence (leakage of urine). Different women have different patterns of incontinence: Some women have difficulty holding back their urine when they hear running water; others lose urine during intercourse or when they cough, sneeze, or lift heavy objects. Although the causes of incontinence increase as people age, the loss of urine is not a normal condition at any age. It can cause emotional distress. Some women can become depressed, and it can cause physical problems like skin infections.
Understanding the type of incontinence and its treatment options can help women ask the right questions and select the best treatment.

4.2. Pelvic Pressure or Pain

While some women are able to go about their daily lives as they had before developing prolapse, others may struggle with new symptoms affecting their quality of life. Physical symptoms can cause a significant amount of distress, as prolapse interferes with normal lifestyle habits such as exercise, socializing, and other cultural practices. Women should seek medical advice and management if their symptoms are starting to affect their families, work, or quality of life. If left untreated, prolapse symptoms can progress and worsen over time.

One of the symptoms associated with bladder wall prolapse, occurring when the connective tissue separating the bladder from the vagina weakens, is pelvic pressure or pain. Additionally, you may notice a worsening of symptoms when coughing, lifting, or sneezing due to increased intra-abdominal pressure. This symptom is likely experienced as a consequence of the heavy, bulging sensation associated with prolapse. In some instances, this discomfort can be accompanied by the feeling of something "falling" down or out of the vagina alongside a sensation of vaginal fullness. This is likely a result of bladder wall prolapse interfering with vaginal function (leading to difficulty urinating, painful intercourse, or tampon placement). In many women who have bladder wall prolapse, symptoms will be mild and can be managed or improved without intervention. While some signs and symptoms associated with prolapse are well known, it is unknown why some patients with prolapse are symptomatic and others are not. It is likely that a combination of prolapse severity, prolapse location, physical attributes, and psychological and socio-cultural factors contribute to perceived symptoms. Symptoms may also be transient and come and go over time.

4.3. Visible Bulge in the Vagina

There are several different structures within the pelvis that can shift down and create a bulge in the vagina. Based on a study published in 1999, about 40% of the bulges identified in the vagina are caused by prolapse affecting the bladder. This is known as cystocele or bladder prolapse. A cystocele is a female pelvic organ prolapse in which the supportive tissues separating the bladder and the vagina weaken, allowing the tissues to stretch, become thin, and sometimes tear. In the process, the muscles resulting in this vaginal wall bulge open (the anterior vaginal wall) and allow the back part of the urinary bladder to physically (and visibly) travel into the vagina. The difference between a typical vaginal bulge (cystocele) and an advanced cystocele is the amount of shifting of the bladder into the vagina.

Another symptom that can indicate a progression of bladder prolapse is the presence of a bulge in the vagina. Most women will experience the sensation of a lump or bulge in the vagina at some point during their lifetime. This is typically a sign that part of the front or back vaginal wall (or both) has shifted from its usual position. A lump in the vagina may be so mild that it is barely noticeable, or it may feel like something is actively falling out of the vagina. The mere sensation of a bulge in the vagina can be disconcerting, causing many women to seek a healthcare evaluation. This decision can be particularly difficult with regard to a bulge in the vagina because many women feel embarrassed or even ashamed about this problem. The presence of a bulge in the vagina can also take a significant emotional toll on many women and decrease their overall quality of life.

5. Diagnosis of Bladder Prolapse

Fluoroscopy: It helps determine the capacity of the bladder such as urinary flow and Pdet. It determines the origin of bladder exit obstruction. Cystography: It helps assess the capacity of the detrusor and helps establish the type of bladder atonia. In addition to being a way to make a diagnosis, cystography also has therapeutic properties, as it helps with a detoxification process of the bladder mucosa. Cystoscopy: It is used to make the diagnosis for doubtful cases. In rare situations, dynamic studies of the urine have been recommended to locate the bladder outlet. These dynamic imaging studies can be performed using different diagnostic methods such as ultrasound, MRI, fluoroscopy, and isotope method.

The diagnosis of bladder prolapse through other imaging tests is done in cases of suspected other pathologies. The imaging techniques used for the evaluation include:

The physical examination is said to be necessary for the diagnosis of mild cases of bladder prolapse. In this, the position of the vagina, bladder, and uterus is determined. Diagnosis of bladder prolapse can also be made through a rectovaginal examination, which is conducted to determine the anterior, posterior, and apical prolapse. This type of examination provides assessment of the apical support.

5.1. Physical Examination

The size of the prolapse is determined in this way. Prolapse of the first and second degree can be difficult to distinguish from one another without ultrasound because in both cases the size of the uterus can look deep in the vagina. The patient's bladder is checked and an ultrasound can be performed. A rectovaginal exam is the insertion of two or more gloved fingers into the vagina and of two or more gloves in the rectum. Care must be taken not to scratch the walls of the vagina or rectum. A rectal exam is used to exclude the posterior wall of the vagina in prolapsed patients. The most common form of prolapse is the formation of the uterus. Therefore, it is important not only to consider the treatment or prevention of bladder prolapse, but also to use diagnostic techniques to examine the presence of the uterus.

The patient should always begin the examination in the lithotomy position. This is the highest position of the table. The hips are at the very edge of the table and the buttocks almost over the end. The lithotomy position allows better access to the inside of the uterus for vaginal examination and allows better access to the inside of the abdomen. There are two types of vaginal examinations: bimanual and speculum. The doctor will use this to determine the position of the uterus and to determine whether a prolapse is located. Most of the time a prolapse hangs near the bottom of the vagina. It is important to remember that the presence of a prolapse only becomes uncomfortable if it breaks into the peritoneum or into the air.

5.2. Imaging Tests

The most commonly performed imaging tests on the human urinary tract are plain film x-rays, which provide a picture using radiation, and/or magnetic resonance imaging (MRI). Both x-rays and MRI tests for women with bladder prolapses look for the presence of urine in the vagina. If this leakage of urine is not present, the bladder prolapse may be less severe. The grading of the severity of bladder prolapse on these studies may also be indicative of potential surgical success, although long-term studies need to be done for confirmation. MRI places the patient inside of a large tube-shaped machine and provides very detailed images. The MRI does not utilize radiation. Evaluation with MRI for bladder prolapse, on the part of the pelvis and usually to be used in combination with imaging your urinary system, should be made by a radiologist with experience in interpreting MRI. Other imaging tests that are not essential for most patients will be available in the future, such as ultrasound and various imaging contrast studies.

The first step in diagnosing a prolapsed bladder is for a healthcare provider to take a patient's medical history. A medical history can provide information about possible risk factors, like pregnancy, childbirth, previous surgeries, lifestyle, and any relevant medical issues. Bladder prolapses are generally diagnosed with a pelvic exam for women. Imaging tests can help to elaborate and quantify the severity of the bladder prolapse. These tests can also help if a surgeon is considering repairing the bladder with surgery. A healthcare provider and/or a radiologist may conduct the test. The patient may receive a scheduling appointment for the test or need to schedule it personally. The intention of any imaging test is to look at the structures between the vaginal and urinary tracts, as well as the urinary system and surrounding organs to evaluate the potential for successful bladder repair. These tests are not always necessary in every patient.

Bladder prolapses generally are diagnosed through a combination of a patient's symptoms and a physical pelvic examination. Imaging tests can be helpful, however, to provide a better understanding of the degree of prolapse and to help in surgical planning.

6. Treatment Options for Bladder Prolapse

Non-surgical options: Conservative options for women include not removing the prolapse, as was seen in the Woman's Priority Study, which investigated the impact of prolapse repair on prolapse symptoms and QoL versus no prolapse repair. Relieving the cystocele symptoms and potentially undiagnosed SUI symptoms can also involve the use of pelvic floor exercises (Kegel exercises) in which the woman is asked to squeeze the muscles that control urine flow, the most robust evidence available to suggest that these exercises reduce prolapse symptoms/severity and cystometric measures is for a contraceptive device (the Continence Ring, Urogynaecology Solutions, Australia). Another form of non-removal involves the use of a pessary device, which are stiff or soft ring-shaped devices which are worn in the vagina to help bridge the weakened areas and provide symptomatic relief, they work on the same principles as a good pelvic floor muscle draw, and therefore, the woman will get a sense of what a pessary can do for her before inserting one.

A range of treatment options exists for bladder prolapse, which encompasses both conservative management and surgical repair. Due to both mixed and low-quality evidence, it is important for women to be aware of all of the treatment options that exist prior to deciding which options they would prefer. It is important to first consider the woman's symptomatology, and then a clinician can provide all appropriate options of management to the woman, with the best evidence base to guide her in her choices. In some countries, clinical guidelines suggest that all women who have been diagnosed with POP should be referred to specialist care for an opinion, to discuss the range of treatment options. It is also important that clinicians are aware of the recommendations 7.3 and 7.4 of the WHO Reproductive Atlas (2004) which indicated that, due to low evidence, it was not possible to recommend surgical repair over no treatment or pessary.

6.1. Conservative Management

Conservative management is based on the relief and control of the symptoms, such as a lump or a bulging mass, a feeling of something coming down or out through the vagina, increased frequency or urgency of urination with or without loss of urine, difficulty voiding or incomplete voiding, pelvic pain or discomfort, low back pain, problems during sexual intercourse, constipation, and fecal incontinence. The nonpharmacologic treatment of pelvic organ prolapse mainly consists of lifestyle modifications. There are several strategies of lifestyle modification available in the conservative management of bladder prolapse. Lifestyle modification and treatment of exacerbated physical activities and constipation may complement or even replace physical therapy in the treatment of prolapse. Dietary counseling and weight reduction are necessary for obese patients. Exercises, such as proper lifting, decreasing time spent on activities that involve straining and heavy work, avoiding afternoon tea or coffee, and drinking water during the day, may be beneficial to all patients. For patients with constipation, good daily hydration, increased physical activity, and a diet rich in fiber are recommended. Biofeedback with pelvic floor re-education is sometimes necessary and successful in controlling constipation while reducing symptoms of prolapse. Some studies have also suggested advising patients to adopt regular timed evacuations. Brashears have recommended the St. Mark's three-month planner to patients with rectocele.

Although a definitive causative relationship cannot be made, many surgical cases of pelvic organ prolapse can be attributed to a failure of conservative management. As transmission of abdominal pressure is the major contributor to pelvic organ support, using non-invasive or low-invasive approaches, such as lifestyle, behavioral, and modification of the daily habits, is of utmost importance in the management of all forms and stages of pelvic organ prolapse.

6.2. Pelvic Floor Exercises (Kegels)

These exercises should be done up to five times a day, for as long as the person believes they are useful to them. It may be necessary to avoid coughing, sneezing, heavy lifting, or standing for long periods until prolapse symptoms improve. Also, do not perform these exercises when urinating because it could strain the bladder. If symptoms worsen or are not relieved, seek advice from a physiotherapist who is specialized in women's wellness.

First, identify the right muscles. When urinating, briefly halt the urine flow or "hold back gas." Those are some of the muscles that you would want to exercise. Next, place one or two fingers inside your vagina. Squeeze as though you're trying not to pass gas or trying to quit peeing. Keep squeezing as you count to 10. Rest for three seconds, then repeat ten times. Exercise with the aim of developing a 10-second contraction that you can perform ten times in a row. Try to keep your buttocks, legs, and abdominal muscles relaxed.

C) Pelvic floor exercises (Kegels): The muscles that support the pelvic organs (also called the "levator muscles") can be impaired, leading to prolapse. Pelvic floor, or Kegel, exercises strengthen them. They can also soothe over-tensioned muscles, relax "bearing-down" muscles, and reduce symptoms. The longer the pelvic organ prolapse, the "looser" these levator muscles tend to get. To do these exercises, adopt the following steps.

6.3. Pessaries

Vaginal pessaries act to support the vaginal wall in the presence of prolapse and thus diminish symptoms of either bulging in the vagina or a vaginal lump. Pessaries are used to relieve symptoms of pelvic organ prolapse and for that reason treatment is entirely symptomatic. The commonest presenting symptom of prolapse is a feeling of something coming down in the vagina, associated with backache, heaviness, aching or pain in the lower abdominal area, urinary and/or fecal incontinence and difficulty with urination or defecation. Prolapse can result in considerable discomfort, irritability and limitation of activities backing its anatomical severity. A psychological element may also be present as a result of sexual dysfunction. Unblocking the urethra and relieving retention using catheterization in cases where there is continued difficulty in voiding or total inability to void.

Pessaries were developed to alleviate the symptoms of pelvic organ prolapse and are available in a variety of shapes and sizes. Identifying the correct size and style of pessary determines the function of the device, the extent of the support it places under the prolapsed vaginal wall, and the degree of symptom relief. The benefit of pessary use is that it offers a non-surgical alternative in women either unfit or non-consenting to surgical repair, although a surgical repair offers the better anatomical correction in the longer term.

6.4. Surgical Interventions

The goal of any surgical procedure for bladder prolapse or vaginal wall data is to improve patients' quality of life, self-esteem, and anatomic support. It is critically important that the indications are clearly established in a broad format. The most fundamental question is whether the patient is willing to accept the risks of the procedure. A comprehensive counseling of the patient with regard to the indications, benefits, and risks of surgery is an important aspect of the management of bladder prolapse. There are a number of surgical interventions available for the management of bladder prolapses including alignment of the bulging anterior vaginal wall and correction of concomitant urinary incontinence.

Cystocele (bladder prolapse) can be surgically corrected if its symptoms are severe enough to affect a woman's quality of life. If a woman is not bothered by vaginal bulging and does not have difficulties with urination, defecation, backache, or pelvic pressure and pain, cystocele can be followed closely without any treatment. It is important to note that surgical correction of cystocele is not designed to last a lifetime and not all cystoceles are symptomatic. Little is known about the appropriate indications for surgical correction because some women may have significant cystoceles that are without symptoms. It is important to understand the effectiveness, benefits, and outcome of surgical intervention for bladder prolapse before a person makes a decision about whether or not to pursue surgical intervention.

7. Prevention Strategies for Bladder Prolapse

1. Maintain a healthy weight. 2. Strictly avoid activities that typically increase abdominal pressure and weaken the pelvic floor, such as heavy lifting, constipation or chronic cough (i.e., cigarette smoking). 3. Change daily habits to regulate bowel movements and avoid chronic constipation. This may mean eating more high-fiber or high-bulk foods and increasing your water intake. 4. Promote good posture and body mechanics with daily activities, including practicing Kegel exercises. 5. Modify eating habits and food intake to avoid straining with bowel movements. You can often decrease dietary irritants, such as bladder irritants, to further encourage bladder health. 6. When moving your bowels, avoid excessive straining and prolonged sitting on the toilet. 7. Practice good daily hygiene with urinary or fecal incontinence. Promptly clean soiled skin, protect from chafing, and manage any issues with your doctor or pediatrician.

There are many strategies that can be employed to reduce your risk of bladder prolapse. Limiting any factors that contribute to weakness in the pelvic floor can help. Some changes or decisions can be made early in life, while others, such as diet and exercise changes, are appropriate at any age. It is important to note that not all women with a history of these factors will develop bladder prolapse. However, some women will have many of these factors without experiencing any other problems.

7.1. Maintaining a Healthy Weight

This added pressure can make it difficult to empty the bladder. If you have had bladder prolapse surgery, it's especially important to keep off extra weight as the condition is more likely to return. Maintaining a healthy weight can be done by eating a balanced diet and exercising on a regular basis. If you are overweight or obese, even just losing a small amount of weight can make a significant difference. Physical activity can help shrink belly fat and fat overall, build muscle strength and support the pelvic organs, increase endurance, and help to maintain a healthy weight. Exercises that strengthen the pelvic floor muscles can also help prevent bladder prolapse. Furthermore, smoking, chronic coughing, and excessive lower body exercise, as previously mentioned, can weaken the pelvic floor support muscle and be predictors of bladder prolapse.

Although aging is the most common cause of bladder prolapse, a few lifestyle modifications can be made to reduce the risk of developing a weakened pelvic floor or incorporating treatments that may help you avoid developing severe cases of the prolapse. One such modification is maintaining a healthy weight. When we carry around excess weight, it puts unnecessary pressure on the pelvic floor. The weak pelvic floor muscles may then become insufficient at supporting the pelvic organs. If this occurs, a pelvic organ prolapse, such as bladder prolapse or cystocele, may develop. Additionally, larger amounts of belly fat can contribute to bladder prolapse. The added weight of belly fat can weaken your pelvic floor muscles while simultaneously pressing against your bladder and pushing it down into the vagina.

Section 7.1: Maintaining a Healthy Weight

7.2. Avoiding Heavy Lifting

You might assume women prone to bladder prolapse can stick to the guidelines of not lifting greater than 2.26 kg or 5 lbs to decrease hip, spine, and pelvic floor disorder risk. But doing so is not the full-term answer for prevention. It was logical to support that the extra weight is more demanding, especially with lifting mechanics. Individual's safer lifting capacity, not to have significant intra-abdominal pressure increases than bringing a safe lifting extent. We assume that it will be especially valid with inclining forward lifting mechanics.

We know that if you have bladder prolapse risk factors, heavy lifting increases your risk of bladder prolapse. We also know that techniques for proper lifting, while reducing the negative impact of heavy lifting on the pelvic floor, cannot take stressors entirely off the pelvic floor. So, lifting nothing heavier than a gallon of milk is commonly suggested, although this is an assumption based on what we know about intra-abdominal pressures when lifting, paired with what is known about heavy lifting when it comes to pelvic organ prolapse. Still, Frances M. and Jeannette T. had dreams and aspirations that could not be easily accomplished without some lifting. Furthermore, Frances M. experienced bladder prolapse despite never lifting anything heavy.

7.3. Proper Posture and Body Mechanics

Understanding the anatomical position of the pelvic organs in the body is helpful in reducing the occurrence of POP. One's body awareness can be helpful in managing their condition. A physical therapist can help with this. A person can start out in a sitting or standing position. Normally, the coccyx will be posterior and inferior. The ASIS (anterior superior iliac spine) and pubic symphysis lie in the same vertical plane. If one has a prolapse or is at risk for a prolapse, there will be a posterior tilt. Think of it as a string tied from the tailbone to a wall, if pulled taut, the body will be in the correct position. This can be done lying down as well and should take place during exercising. Focusing attention on pelvic tilt and proper posture while working out can retrain the body.

Maintaining a good posture can help to prevent an increase in intra-abdominal pressure. When the body is out of alignment, the organs are less supported and can push on the pelvic floor. Once out of alignment, movement can magnify the pressure on the pelvic floor. By preventing the malalignment and decreasing the pressure on the pelvic floor, a person may experience less occurrence of POP (Prolapsed Organs of the Pelvic Floor). In practice, many people find that during a visit with a physical therapist, a simple correction of posture results in the lessening of the prolapse. Instructing the patient as to the biomechanics of prolapse prevention is beneficial, as it can put the patient in control of their prolapse management.

8. Outlook and Prognosis

Furthermore, complications are also reported, although they do not occur frequently. When evaluating the outcomes of pelvic organ prolapse, sexual disorders have only been assessed in a minority of studies. They range between 15% and 82% for improved sexual life (2-point change), 17%–42% for improved satisfaction with coitus (1-point change), 60%–62% reporting painless intercourse, and 22%–57% to be sexually active reduction in nodes-incidence after ring pessaries. Success rates range from 97% to 99.7%. With respect to functional outcomes (concomitant complaints), sexual outcomes have been assessed in very few studies. Failure rates in operation based on reduction of incontinence due to the operation have only been presented in publications by Lensen 2001, Costantini 2004, and Schmid 2005 and only with operations with concomitant support of the proximal urethra. They range between 11% and 20%. Complications are moderate and generally not severe and range between 7.9% and 13.2%. Several studies over the medium term (less than 24 months) show high satisfaction rates of 91%–93%.

If a bladder prolapse remains untreated, it can continue to progress in size and severity, although the rate of progression may vary. Next to a worsening of symptoms and a further decrease in quality of life, long-term bladder prolapse can cause increasing problems. For example, it can lead to chronic urinary tract infections. However, the development of incontinence as well as other complaints, such as defecation disorders and/or sexual disorders, caused by further pelvic organ descent needs to be anticipated individually. Symptoms themselves may improve with behavioral or mechanical modifications but generally will not resolve nor improve in severity. However, data on the progression of prolapse without any treatment over long periods of time are scarce. Regarding vaginal pessaries, success rates between 39.3% and 90% after one year are reported for vaginal pessaries with different forms and followed for up to 12 months. Incontinence may worsen in up to 1.8%.

8.1. Prognosis of Untreated Bladder Prolapse

It is not clear as to what extent untreated bladder prolapse can produce de novo or worsen lower urinary tract symptoms and it has not been possible to come to an agreement. It makes logical sense that treatment of prolapse, whether medical or surgical, should be considered once recordings affirm that it is a likely cause of the symptoms and verify improved outcomes. The diagnosis of bladder prolapse depends mainly on a detailed history, pelvic examination, and parametric ultrasonography. Therefore, the true prevalence of bladder prolapse among women with pelvic floor disorder is not well described.

Section 8.1 Prognosis of untreated bladder prolapse: Over time, the opening at the proximal end of the prolapsed bladder may enlarge, leading to complete exposure and protrusion of the prolapsed bladder. The vaginal epithelium may become injured and inflamed, leading to inflammation of the surrounding tissue that may become trapped in the rectocele, or the modifications in vaginal capacitive receptors might induce a sensation of protrusion or prominent roadmap. Aside from the bothersome symptoms, prolapsed anterior vaginal wall and bladder might lead to complications such as hydronephrosis or post-void residual urine volume, which may in turn result in recurrent urinary tract infection and renal impairment. Untreated bladder prolapse may result in reduced quality of life and social participation, which may pose a mental health danger. Furthermore, women with anterior vaginal wall prolapse have a greater risk of pelvic organ prolapse after surgical treatment.

8.2. Success Rates of Treatment Options

There is a paucity of published data regarding the treatment of bladder prolapse; research is scant and evidence-based management plans are lacking. The optimal management is uncertain. We thank Dr. Husain for the opportunity to clarify our viewpoint. We agree with her observation that anterior colporrhaphy has high success rates when performed correctly in appropriately selected patients. It can, however, be challenging to predict the likelihood of failure. If the supportive tissues of the bladder are good, with evidence of prolapse due to an isolated area of weakness in the anterior vaginal wall and minimal or controlled stress incontinence, there may still be a place for colporrhaphy. Moreover, women who are committed to a non-operative approach may choose to have an initial vaginal repair. Optimized success rates (mean 82.6%, range 65-94%) are achieved when a synthetic mesh is incorporated into the repair to augment weak native tissue; other methods of reinforcing the tissue have lower mean reported success rates (74%) for treating stages 2-4 disease. Mitigation of the relative risk of recurrent prolapse after surgery to treat anterior vaginal wall prolapse should focus on optimizing the choice of treatment to the individual patient. Treatment after failure can be successful and should be undertaken regardless of the prior procedure she had.

Success rates for anterior repair surgery for bladder prolapse can range from 70-90%. However, women have a slight risk of the prolapse recurring over time. In approximately 8-25% of cases, the anterior wall prolapse will reoccur. There are no long-term studies on success rates of vaginal vault suspension surgery. However, estimates suggest that the success rate may range from 60-90%. The success rates for perineal body reconstruction are estimated to be between 90-100%.